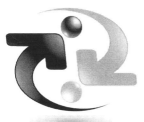

how2become
A Nail Technician

By Philippa Oakley

If you're interested in the
techniques, have a creativ
interest in working with
consider a career as

D0857569

OLDHAM LIBRARIES

3 470 783 5

Orders: Please contact How2become Ltd, Suite 2, 50 Churchill Square Business Centre, Kings Hill, Kent ME19 4YU.

You can order via the e-mail address info@how2become.co.uk or through Gardners Books at Gardners.com

ISBN: 9781907558450

Copyright © 2012 Philippa Oakley. All rights reserved.

All rights reserved. Apart from any permitted use under UK copyright law, no part of this publication may be reproduced or transmitted in any form or by any means, electronic or mechanical, including photocopying, recording, or any information, storage or retrieval system, without permission in writing from the publisher or under licence from the Copyright Licensing Agency Limited. Further details of such licenses (for reprographic reproduction) may be obtained from the Copyright Licensing Agency Ltd, Saffron House, 6-10 Kirby Street, London EC1N 8TS.

Typeset for How2become Ltd by Molly Hill, Canada.

Printed in Great Britain for How2become Ltd by:
CMP (uk) Limited, Poole, Dorset.

CONTENTS

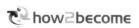

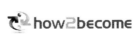

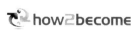

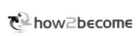

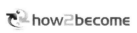

The information contained in this document is for information and instruction only.

The owner/publisher cannot accept any responsibility for the level of success achieved or gained by individuals or parties acting upon information contained in this book. It is down to the individual/s efforts and application.

The owner/publisher and copyright holder accept no responsibility whatsoever for any claim/s originating from use or misuse of the information, application, execution or products and procedures described within or on any part or part of the buyer.

First published 2012

Copyright © Philippa Oakley. All rights reserved.

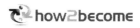 how2become

CHAPTER ONE

WHAT IS A NAIL TECHNICIAN?

If you often find yourself admiring the nails of others, keen to know about the latest nail trends and techniques and have a genuine interest in working with people, then a career as a nail technician could be just right for you.

Maybe you are considering which career path to take. It could be that you already work in the beauty industry and wish to expand your skills, or perhaps you are looking for a work-life balance that can offer the flexibility you need in your life right now. A career as a nail technician offers a range of benefits to meet almost all lifestyles.

But what does a nail technician actually do and how do you become one?

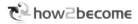

A nail technician is a trained professional working in the health and beauty industry who works to take care of, decorate and improve a client's nails. Nail technicians perform manicures – dealing with the nails on the hands, and pedicures – dealing with the nails on the feet. Most nail technicians also offer hand or foot massages as part of their treatments.

A nail technician does not just shape and decorate a client's nails – they are also responsible for the health of their client's nails as well. A nail technician must also be able to prepare nails for specialist treatments and perform such treatments as: extensions, adding gemstones, adding acrylic nails, glitter, air-brushing techniques, stencilled patterns and also be able to maintain existing treatments or replace nails.

An important aspect of the role of a nail technician is to be able to advise their client on suitable after-care for their nails too.

Nail technicians work either in salons, spas, health clubs, on cruise ships, in holiday resorts, in hotels, in department stores, from their own homes or offer a mobile service.

WHY BECOME A NAIL TECHNICIAN?

"I became a nail technician to gain a profession that would enable me to either become self employed or employed within a salon setting." Jo Cura, Nail technician, Beauty Therapist, and College Lecturer.

"I became a nail technician purely by chance. I was made redundant from my current job at the time, and I saw a job advertised at the Job Centre for a manicurist. I thought, I could do that as I had previously taken a 6 week manicure and pedicure course at Luton and Dunstable College (not because I wanted to do it for a job – just so I knew what I was doing on myself)." Emma Briers, home-based nail technician.

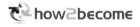

"I had my nails done for my wedding in 1991, which I continued with for a couple of years. In 1995 my nail tech decided she couldn't do the Selby area any more as she was so busy in York. She suggested I went on a course as I always had them prepped and shaped before she arrived." Isabella, home-based nail technician since 1995.

Despite the recent recession, one area which hasn't suffered has been the health and beauty sector, in fact it is growing!

A manicure or a pedicure is an affordable treat and people like to treat themselves, especially in a recession. It makes them feel good and look good. It is a pampering treatment that most people can afford.

Demand for nail technicians is growing. A recent report by Local Data Support, a research company, shows that nail bars are the fastest growing sector on the high street, making up 16.5% of all new high street stores in the past three years.

Thea Green started up Nails Inc in 2009 and it is now the largest chain of nail bars in the UK with a turnover of £25 million. In an interview with the Daily Mail on 31 January 2012 she said: *"Nail salons have enduring appeal as they are a fast and affordable way to feel groomed. People are working so hard and under an increased amount of pressure, so taking 15 minutes of 'me' time makes them feel pampered."*

"After visiting a nail salon, customers are likely to receive compliments and then often feel positive and confident about themselves. Nail salons have the feel-good factor and a manicure isn't as drastic as a haircut or other beauty treatments."

It is currently estimated that there over 17,000 businesses in the UK employing nail technicians. Many nail technicians each year leave salons and spas etc to set up their own

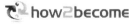

mobile nail service. There always seems to be job vacancies for nail technicians.

A nail technician in the UK can expect to earn between £12,000 and £20,000 a year, with the most experienced technicians earning around £25,000 or more.

As a nail technician you have the flexibility to work when and where you choose. You can work in a salon or a spa, on a cruise ship, in a gym or you can set up on your own. Many nail technicians also go on to teach at colleges, like Jo Cura, or in beauty salons. Others work exclusively in the fashion industry, maintaining models' hands for photo shoots or working in television and theatre.

It is an incredibly flexible career and has no age barriers to entry. Many people become nail technicians as a second or third career. It can be studied either full-time in as little as a week, or part-time. You can study at home or at a college.

Both the studying and the job itself easily fit in around school hours or around other careers. It is a skill that can be learned relatively quickly and one where you can soon earn back the fees from your course.

To help you, think about what your motivations are for considering a new career as a nail technician. Are you looking for a part time job that will fit around the needs of your family? Perhaps you are hoping to travel. Maybe you would like to enter the health and beauty profession, but you are not absolutely sure it is the right move for you, so training as a nail technician would be a good starting point? Keep these motivations clear in your mind, as these will form the basis of the type of training that will be most suited to you to start your new career.

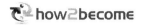

WHAT DO NAIL TECHNICIANS DO?

Nail technicians are health and beauty professionals who are responsible for the clients' nails. In general this can be split into four main areas:

- Health and Safety of Clients
- Manicure
- Pedicure
- Nail Artistry

Health and Safety of Clients

As a nail technician you are responsible for the health and safety of your clients whether you are treating them in a salon, your home or their home. You need to keep all your equipment clean and sterilize equipment regularly.

You will also need to check the health and condition of your client's nails and advise on appropriate after-care.

You will be using a wide variety of chemicals in your work and you need to ensure these are stored safely.

Manicures

There is much more to a manicure than filing down nails and applying polish! Manicure comes from the Latin words for hand (manus) and care (cura). It is literally 'care of the hands' – not just of the nails.

A manicure involves filing and shaping the nails, removing cuticles, applying softening lotions and treatment oils, massaging the hands, and applying nail polish or nail treatments.

It is thought that the first manicures were performed over 5000 years ago! In ancient India henna was applied to

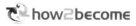

the nails as a polish. Around 4000 years ago in Babylonia, manicure tools were created out of gold to keep nails looking trim and healthy. The first nail polish was developed in China around 3000 years ago! Only the wealthy and important people could afford nail polish and so a manicured hand was a signal of your status in society!

In ancient Egypt, Cleopatra apparently preferred to have red nails whilst both Roman and Egyptian military commanders regularly painted their nails to match the colours they were wearing.

In the 18th Century the French manicure was developed in Paris. A French manicure is a technique whereby pink and white nail polishes are applied to make the nails look natural, but better than natural nails. French manicures became incredibly popular in the 1920s and 1930s but are still a popular choice today.

When performing a manicure today a nail technician will first of all analyze the condition of her client's nails. Nails are made from keratin, which is the same substance your body uses to create hair and the top layer of your skin, and as such, can be damaged by certain treatments or chemicals. A nail technician needs to assess the 'health' of a client's nails before deciding on the best course of treatment.

Then a nail technician will usually begin by removing the cuticle and then applying lotions or oils to improve the condition of the nail bed.

More lotions are usually applied to the hand and a hand massage given.

Then any filing or shaping is carried out before nail treatments – nail polish etc, is applied.

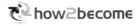

A manicure can last anywhere from 15 minutes for a quick "paint and tidy" to an hour for a full treatment.

Pedicures

Just as manicure means care of the hands, pedicure means care of the feet. Pedicures have been performed as long as manicures, from what we can gather. There is, for example, pictures depicting a pedicure in some Egyptian tombs.

A pedicure is always a longer procedure than a manicure, lasting at least 45 minutes, and is viewed by the client as more of a pampering experience.

A pedicure involves removing rough skin from the bottom of the foot, shaping nails and applying treatments. A pedicure always involves a foot soak and a massage.

Usually the treatment begins with a foot soak in warm water to which a cleaning agent has been added.

The nail technician works on one foot at a time. It is usual to leave one foot in the footbath whilst drying the other and using a pumice stone or electric foot softener to remove hard skin from the foot.

Then this foot is massaged with lotions and left on a towel whilst the nail technician handles the other foot.

Then the nails are filed and trimmed and treated as required

Nail Artistry

Whereas ten years ago the most you could hope for from a manicure was a nice shade of nail polish or maybe a French manicure, now with skilled nail artists the only limit to what you can do with your nails is your imagination. Today's nail technicians need to be creative! Most customers no longer just want beautifully painted nails, but want artistic designs.

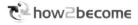

As a nail artist you could be applying gemstones, 3D designs, airbrushing designs onto nails or painting designs free hand.

If you have an artistic temperament this is ideal for you. If not, then thankfully, most skills, such as gemstones and air-brushing can be learned.

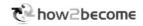

CHAPTER TWO

TYPES OF TREATMENTS OFFERED BY A NAIL TECHNICIAN

As a qualified nail technician you will be expected to offer most of the following treatments either in a salon or in your client's home.

- Shape & Polish
- Tidy &Trim
- Basic Manicure
- French Manicure
- Japanese Manicure
- Hot Oil Manicures
- Paraffin Dips
- Gel Nail Manicures
- Basic Pedicures

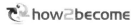

- Luxury Pedicures
- Gel Nail Pedicures
- Nail Extensions
- Acrylic Tips
- Gel Overlays
- Gemstones
- Airbrush Designs

You won't be expected to do them all straight away! You will learn how to do each treatment and practise a lot before you gain your qualification. Some skills, such as free-hand nail art, are only learned after becoming qualified.

Before doing any treatment, you will ALWAYS check the condition of your client's nails and only proceed with a treatment if appropriate. You will learn more about this on your courses and in salons.

Let's take a brief look at each of these treatments.

SHAPE & POLISH

This is the basic manicure that lasts fifteen minutes at most and is the most requested treatment in nail bars across the country. As a nail technician you simply file the nails and apply a coat of polish.

TRIM & TIDY

This is the male version of the above. Many men, businessmen in particular, are becoming more aware of the condition of their nails and hands and want them to look their best. A trim and tidy is a very quick treatment, involving trimming and filing nails and buffing them to give them a natural, healthy shine.

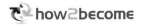

BASIC MANICURE

One step up from these treatments, a basic manicure involves cuticle care, some massaging of the hands, applying lotions and oils to the hands and nail beds, filing and shaping and then applying a polish.

FRENCH MANICURE

This is quite involved and costs more than a basic manicure. After treating the cuticles and shaping the nails a series of nail polishes are applied to the nails to make them look natural, but better than natural. This is a highly skilled task and one you will need to practice a lot! People who want French manicures want exquisite, perfect looking nails.

JAPANESE MANICURE

This involves treating the cuticles and shaping the nails and then using a variety of buffing and polishing techniques to create a natural, polished look on the nails without actually using any polish.

HOT OIL MANICURES

These are used when the client's nails are brittle, dry or ridged or where the cuticles are damaged. By using hot oils the nail bed can absorb more of the oils and be in a much better state by the end of the treatment. You heat up olive oil or a mineral oil in an electric oil heater. At the point in a normal manicure where you would place the client's nails in a bowl of warm water, you place them in the hot oil. Then you massage the hot oil into your client's fingers and nails. Dry off and complete the manicure as normal.

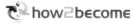

PARAFFIN DIPS

Once seen as a luxury only offered by a few exclusive salons, paraffin dips are becoming an incredibly popular treatment. Paraffin dips leave hands incredibly smooth. A paraffin dip involves dipping the hand (or foot) into a bath of melted paraffin, removing it, re-dipping it four or five times until the hand is fully covered in paraffin.

Wrap the hand/food in Clingfilm or a plastic bag and a towel or a mitt. Leave for ten minutes, remove the wrappings and massage the hand.

Now continue with the manicure as normal but dehydrate the nail beds before applying polish.

GEL NAIL MANICURES

These manicures involve coating the nails with a soak-off gel treatment that can be coloured or in the style of a French manicure, but which allows the nail underneath to grow. It is considered healthier for the nail than normal acrylic extensions or tips. These manicures are recommended for clients with bitten or broken nails.

LUXURY MANICURES

These involve normal manicure procedures as well as a hand massage or treatment with either paraffin dips or special oils and lotions.

BASIC PEDICURES

A basic pedicure involves a foot soak, removal of hard and rough skin from the sole of the foot, pushing back or removing cuticles, shaping nails and applying a nail polish.

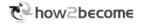

LUXURY PEDICURES

In addition to the steps involved in a basic pedicure, a luxury pedicure includes a foot massage treatment and use of oils or lotions on the feet.

GEL NAIL PEDICURES

As with gel nail manicures, this involves coating the nails with a soak-off gel treatment to make the nails look beautiful whilst allowing the nail underneath to grow. These are suitable for discoloured, broken or problem nails.

NAIL EXTENSIONS

After the manicure, instead of applying polish the nails are prepared for acrylic nail extensions. The nail is scuffed and then special acrylic glue is applied to each nail in turn and an acrylic nail is attached. These are then shaped and painted to the client's requirements – either with normal polish, a French manicure, gemstones, 3D designs, airbrush designs or hand-drawn designs.

ACRYLIC TIPS

These are an alternative to full nail extensions and involve attaching an acrylic tip to the nail to make the nails look longer. These can then be shaped and painted as normal nails.

GEL OVERLAYS

Gel overlays promote natural nail growth and health and can be applied directly to nails or over extensions; they can also

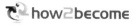

be applied as tips only. Gel overlays strengthen nails and under a UVA lamp dry to a hard, shiny finish. They come in natural or a variety of colours, including French manicure.

GEMSTONES

Gemstones can be stuck onto nails for a fancy effect. They are normally stuck on with a special nail adhesive and then coated with clear polish to protect them from damage and falling off.

AIRBRUSH DESIGNS

By using a miniature air brush the nail technician can create beautiful works of art on each nail. Technicians use stencils to create most of the designs, but some, highly skilled nail technicians use the airbrush to paint their own designs onto the nail – this is known as painting designs free-hand.

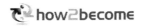

CHAPTER THREE

WHAT DOES IT TAKE TO BE A SUCCESSFUL NAIL TECHNICIAN?

"You have to be patient, dedicated and reliable," said Isabella. "It isn't an easy thing to do; you need practice and to have patience to begin with. You need also to believe in yourself and be positive and praise yourself when praise is required. Try not to be too judgemental with yourself either. Do as much training as you can, keeping up with trends and new products is vital. Go to shows, see what is out there. The nail business is never ending..."

As you can see, there is a lot to the job of being a nail technician; it is varied and creative, incredibly sociable and one that can be done full or part time, and as either employed or self employed. If you are thinking of becoming a nail technician you need to make sure it is a job that will suit you.

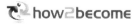

ESSENTIAL SKILLS AND COMPETENCIES OF A NAIL TECHNICIAN

To be a successful nail technician you need to have or to develop the following key skills and competencies.

- Creativity
- People Skills
- Patience
- Attention to detail
- Steady hand – gained through practice and more practice at the nail desk!
- Interest in your own personal development – keeping up to date with the latest trends and techniques
- Organisation Skills
- Admin Skills
- Ability to work on your own
- Ability to work with others
- Diligence

Creativity
You need to be able to visualise what will and won't look good on a client's nails and to be able to come up with and paint appropriate designs onto their nails. You need to be inspired by design and want to create beautiful nails, designs and patterns.

People Skills
You will be working with people all day long – so naturally you need good people skills. This means good communication skills, good listening skills, tact, diplomacy and a friendly, outgoing nature. You must not get angry with your clients or gossip about your clients or fellow members of staff. You

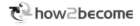

need to be seen to be friendly, knowledgeable, happy and outgoing.

Patience
It can take a long time to perform a manicure or pedicure and even longer to paint intricate designs onto nails, apply extensions, gemstones etc. You must be patient and able to concentrate for long periods of time. You also need to be patient to deal with clients who cannot make up their mind what treatment they want!

Attention to Detail
As a nail technician you need to ensure that the designs you create are perfect; that varnishes look good and that all the nails you create for your client match. You must also ensure you always carry out your manicure and pedicure steps in the right order and never forget a step.

Steady Hand
This really is an essential skill for a nail technician; your clients expect that their nails will look fantastic and you need to be very steady when applying varnishes and designs to ensure they live up to your clients' expectations.

Interest in your own personal development
You must be keen to continue to learn new skills and techniques. You need to continue to take courses and develop the range of service you can offer.

Organisation Skills
As a nail technician you need stellar organisational skills. You need to organise your appointments, allow enough time for treatments etc. You need to ensure your equipment is clean and sterile and you are meeting your health and safety

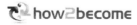

obligations. You need to keep your chemicals safe and secure and fully stocked. You need to keep your polishes, brushes, tips, overlays etc, organised so you can use them when you need to.

Admin Skills

If you are renting a room in a salon, you need to ensure you make your rent payments on time. If you are profit sharing, you need to keep accurate records of what you take. Unless you are employed directly by someone else, a salon or leisure centre as a nail technician you will also need to keep track of your earnings and expenses for tax purposes and ensure your insurance is up to date.

Ability to Work on Your Own

As a nail technician you will be working on your own with the client most of the time. This means you need to be a self-starter who can work happily on your own for long periods of time.

Ability to Work with Others

If you are working in a salon you must also be able to work happily with others and be willing to take over and do other tasks, such things as helping out on reception or tidying up as needed, even if they are not part of your normal duties

Diligence

This is a word we don't often hear these days. Basically it means stickability. As a nail technician you must be prepared to put in the hours needed to perfect your skills. And it does take many, many hours to become a skilled nail technician. You need to do lots of study and even when qualified, you need to take refresher courses to keep up to date with the latest innovations in nail technology.

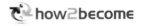

Flexibility

Nail technicians are most in demand when other people are enjoying their leisure time. If you want to succeed as a nail technician you need to be prepared to work unsocial hours such as evenings and weekends.

Also, whilst being a nail technician is not a physically demanding job, it can be strenuous spending so much time bent over other people's hands and feet. If you find this hard, try some stretches and Yoga or Pilates!

Still interested? Great! Then let's look at what you need to study to become a nail technician.

WHAT YOU STUDY TO BECOME A NAIL TECHNICIAN

Nail Technicians study much more than how to apply nail varnish. They also have to learn a lot of science and business skills too.

Regardless of which qualification route you take, to become a nail technician you will need to study:

- Health and safety requirements of a beauty salon
- The anatomy and physiology of the hand and foot
- The anatomy and physiology of the nail
- Nail diseases and disorders
- Skin diseases and disorders
- Bacteriology
- Sterilisation and sanitation of equipment
- Salon reception duties
- Salon appointment duties and client record keeping
- Salon business skills

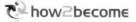

- Manicures
- Pedicures
- Customer service
- How to sell other products/services to clients
- Some nail art techniques (polishes, gels, acrylics, air-brushing) depending on the course studied and at what level it is studied.

FORMAL QUALIFICATIONS REQUIRED TO WORK AS A NAIL TECHNICIAN

Jo, who is a lecturer at a college as well as working in a salon says *"You need to have the NVQ 2 in Nail technology, as a minimum."*

Danielle Cook, who works in a salon and Isabella both agree that the minimum qualification you need is *"Manicure and pedicure training."*

But, as Emma puts it *"Basically, at the moment to be a nail technician, you do not have to have a recognised qualification! However, to make you stand out from the millions of other technicians out there, a qualification or training with a respectable and well known company will help you gain and keep your clients."*

As you can see, there is some disagreement as to what basic qualifications you need to be employed as a nail technician in the UK. However, if you wish to work in a salon, you usually need to have one of the following qualifications:

- NVQ Level 2 Diploma in Nail Services
- NVQ Level 3 Diploma in Nail Services
- CIBTAC Nail Technician Diploma
- BABTAC Nail Technician Diploma

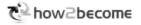

- ITEC Level 2 Certificate in Nail Technology
- ITEC Level 3 Diploma in Nail Technology
- VTCT Level 2 Certificate in Nail Technology
- VTCT Level 3 Diploma in Nail Technology.

Level 2 certificates and diplomas will gain you an entry level position as a junior nail technician. Level 3 will gain you employment as a senior nail technician. We will cover the length of each of these courses and whether you can study full time or part time as we cover each qualification later.

Some colleges will require you to do a course in manicures before progressing onto advanced nail techniques; others cover everything.

You can study these qualifications locally either full or part-time at colleges of further education or private colleges. You can also study to become a nail technician by distant learning methods – again either full or part time. If you choose to study via distance learning you will need to gain several days worth of experience in a nail bar or salon to prove you can do the skills you have learned.

GOING SELF-EMPLOYED?

If you wish to set up in business as a self-employed nail technician, bear in mind you might also need a licence from the environmental health department of your local council. Some councils have minimum qualification requirements they expect nail technicians to have before they grant them a licence. Some will accept any of the above qualifications, whereas others will only accept the NVQ.

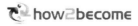

CHAPTER FOUR

HOW TO GET THE QUALIFICATIONS YOU NEED

"I did a 2 day course with Star Nails at Denis William's Hair and Beauty Warehouse in York. The course I did was Silk and Fibreglass. Since then I have done various other courses; CND Acrylics, Ezflow Gels. I've got over 20 certificates now, having done various nail art and design acrylic courses as well as Spa Manicure and Spa Pedicure with Creative, Minx and Shellac courses and Gelish design. And when anything new pops up I look into that too." Says Isabella.

Danielle said *"I did a City & Guilds Level 2 & 3 in Beauty Therapy at College, which gave me my basic manicure training and I have then gone on private courses with various product houses."*

Jo studied a CIBTAC NVQ level 2 & 3 in Beauty Therapy.

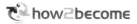 how2become

Whilst Emma said: *"I passed and received my certificate of graduation with Salon System, for Professional Acrylic Nail Extensions, and Fibreglass and Silk Nail Extensions. This was back in January 2003. I then went on to work for a different employer who put me on a Bio Sculpture Gel Nail training course as an apprentice. I can't remember the cost of this course but you will pay around £420 now. This was a two day course and then I went back later to be assessed."*

"Other qualifications I have are a Creative Nail Academy conversion. This is a one day course. I also attended a City and Guilds Beauty Therapy Level 3 course which I had 6 months to complete and had to attend College 1 day each week. I was assessed on my portfolio work and observation. Nail technicians do not have to have this qualification, but it teaches you all about health and safety, consultation techniques, anatomy and physiology, and all about the products and their chemistry. Also it teaches you about client aftercare, which I feel has helped me gain the clients I have today, and given me a better insight into my profession."

As you can see, there are many routes into the nail technician profession.

Some people start as apprentices and learn on the job.

Others start by doing a basic course in manicures, then slowly build up their skills and experience by doing appropriate City & Guild Qualifications in such topics as UV gels or acrylics and learning 'on the job', whereas others take courses at colleges or private colleges.

There is no one 'right' route into the profession; you need to choose the best fit for you, your circumstances, the time you have available and your finances. Let's look at each option in more detail.

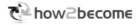

APPRENTICESHIPS

Contrary to popular belief, apprenticeships are not only for the young school leaver. In fact, apprenticeships are open to everyone over the age of 16, whether they have worked before or not. If you want to train in a new career and can find an employer willing to take you on, you can become an apprentice.

There are two levels of apprenticeship offered in Nail Service: an intermediate apprenticeship and an advanced apprenticeship. Apprentices can earn anything from £80 to £170 a week. You can find details of the apprenticeship scheme here:

http://www.apprenticeships.org.uk/Types-of-Apprenticeships/Retail-and-Commercial-Enterprise/Nail-Services.aspx

I suggest you do a Google search as you go through the following details regarding qualifications, local colleges and private organisations, to find the provider nearest to you.

COLLEGE COURSES

Level 2 NVQ in Nail Services
On this course you will gain theoretical and practical knowledge in:

- Anatomy & Physiology of skin, nails, bones, muscles and circulatory systems.
- Manicure
- Pedicure
- Nail Art
- False nails (Fibreglass , Acrylic and Gel nail systems)

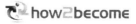

- Health & Safety
- Salon skills and employment standards
- Promoting services and products
- Customer care

Most colleges have salons on site where you will learn and practice your skills.

Level 2 NVQ in Nail Services at Local Colleges
You can study this qualification at many local colleges of further education as well as at a wide variety of private colleges and online.

If you want to enrol at a local college, you will usually need to have a minimum of 4 GCSEs including English.

At a local college this course normally costs around £500 for a 34 week part-time course, with 6 hours study a week. In addition to this you will need to purchase a nail kit (around £150), study books and pay exam fees.

When you study at a college you will get to practice in a fully equipped salon on real people as well as other trainees. In addition to this, most colleges also arrange work experience with local salons too.

Level 2 NVQ at Private Colleges
Some nail institutes and private colleges also offer Level 2 NVQ in Nail Services. With these colleges you can study for the diploma full-time in five weeks. The costs for these courses are around £1,300 plus VAT plus the cost of your nail kit, which varies from college to college.

Private colleges also offer a variety of part-time intensive courses too, some running over several weekends others over a few hours a week. Prices for these courses vary

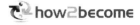

considerably depending upon the speed with which you want to complete the course.

There are no minimum entry requirements at the private colleges. However, depending on where you study, you might need to arrange your own work experience in order to gain the salon hours you need to qualify.

Level 2 NVQ in Nail Services Online

Some online colleges also offer the NVQ Level 2 via a mix of onsite and distance learning. On these courses you will need to find willing volunteers to allow you to practice your skills and whom you can photograph for your portfolio.

Level 3 NVQ in Nail Services

This is the follow-on course from Level 2 and enables you to gain employment as a senior nail technician.

The course consists of 3 mandatory units and a minimum of 4 optional units.

The mandatory units are:

- How to monitor procedures to safely control work operations
- How to enhance and maintain nails using UV gel
- How to enhance and maintain nails using liquid and powder

You then need to choose at least four of the following units:

- How to develop a range of creative nail images
- How to plan and create nail art designs
- How to plan and provide airbrush design for nails
- How to contribute to the financial effectiveness of the business

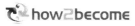

- How to contribute to the planning and implementation of promotional activities
- How to prepare and finish nail overlays using electric files
- How to enhance and maintain nails using wraps

Level 3 NVQ in Nail Services at Local Colleges
To enrol onto the Level 3 course you will have to have completed the Level 2 course.

At local colleges this course costs around £850 – £950 for a 34 week course with 6 hours of study a week. Some colleges offer 1 day or evening a week for 10 weeks. Once again you will need to purchase extra equipment as needed and pay exam fees.

Level 3 NVQ in Nail Services at Private Colleges
You can study the Level 3 course at private colleges and nail institutes. Again, however, you will need to have completed Level 2 first, or a Level 2 in manicure or pedicure services.

Level 3 is usually only available to study part-time or via intensive courses. Costs vary considerably from college to college and from region to region.

CIBTAC and BIBTAC Nail Technician Diploma
These are offered by a variety of private colleges and beauty institutes. Again they can be studied either full time or part-time. To gain access to the course you normally need to have a qualification in manicure.

The costs of these qualifications are around £700 – £900 plus VAT plus nail kits.

These qualifications also require a minimum amount of salon time before you are recognised as qualified.

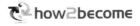

If you have a qualification in manicure, you need to complete 15 hours in a salon environment. If you don't have the manicure qualification, you need to complete 35 hours in a salon environment.

This means you need to find a salon that will allow you to complete your work experience to gain your qualification – most colleges will arrange this for you.

You will also need to spend 15 hours contact time (with clients) at the college based salon (if you have the manicure qualification) and 30 hours if you do not.

The typical course content for these courses is:

- Skin Diseases of the Hands & Feet
- Nail Diseases & Disorders
- Professional Tools & Implements
- Nail Care Products, their composition and uses
- Anatomy of the hands & feet
- Anatomy & Physiology of the Skin
- Sterilisation & Sanitation
- Hygiene & Personal care/safety
- First Aid
- Client Care & Professionalism
- Professional Ethics
- Professional Manicure – Revision
- Professional Pedicure – Revision
- Application of Acrylic Nails (Natural, French. Long, Short)
- Application of Gel Nails (Natural, French. Long, Short)
- Refills, Repairs, Rebalancing

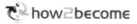

- Removal of False Nails
- Nail Paint / Varnish / Colours / French
- Nail Art & Gems

ITEC Level 2 Certificate in Nail Technology
The ITEC qualification is an internationally recognised version of the NVQ qualification at level 2.

On this course you study:

- Structure of the Nail
- Anatomy and Physiology of hands and feet
- Conditions of hands and feet
- Nail diseases and disorders
- Health and Hygiene
- Gel Nail application
- Acrylic Nail application
- Silk Wraps and Fibre glass
- Gel Toe Nails
- Professional Conduct
- Business Awareness

In the UK you can only study for ITEC Level 2 certificate in Nail Technology at the following locations:

- Nails and Beauty Academy, London
- Sheffield School of Health and Beauty
- White Rose School of Health and Beauty, Barnsley
- Stockport College of Further and Higher Education
- Yorkshire College of Beauty, Leeds

Costs of these courses are around £800. As with the NVQ Level 2, you will normally get to practice on 'real' clients in a

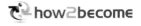

salon in the college or you will have work experience in local salons.

ITEC Level 3 Diploma in Nail Technology

The ITEC qualification is an internationally recognised version of the NVQ qualification at level 3.

On this course you study thirteen mandatory units:

- Provide manicure treatments
- Provide pedicure treatments
- Create an image based on a theme in the hair and beauty sector
- Apply and maintain nail enhancements
- Design and apply nail art
- Airbrush designs for nails
- Enhance nails using electric files
- Monitor and maintain health and safety practice in the salon
- Salon reception duties
- Display stock to promote sales in the salon
- Client care and communication in beauty related industries
- Working in the beauty related industries
- Working with colleagues within beauty related industries

In the UK you can only study for ITEC Level 3 Diploma in Nail Technology at the following locations:

- Nails and Beauty Academy, London
- Sheffield School of Health and Beauty
- White Rose School of Health and Beauty, Barnsley

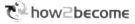

- Stockport College of Further and Higher Education
- Creative Academy + Manchester,
- Central Coll. of Health & Beauty, Leeds
- SAKS Education, Darlington

To progress onto Level 3 you will need to have completed Level 2. The costs of this course are also around £800.

VTCT Level 2 in Nail Technology

For the Level 2 you need to study 4 mandatory units and one optional unit.

The mandatory units are:

- Follow health and safety practice in the salon
- Provide and maintain nail enhancement
- Client care and communication in beauty-related industries
- Provide manicure treatments
- The optional units are:
- Provide pedicure treatments
- Provide Nail Art

You can study this qualification at many local colleges and private colleges. It is normally taught part-time over one evening a week for 24 weeks in local colleges and over a shorter, more intensive period in private colleges and beauty institutes.

There are no entry requirements for this course. The costs of this course vary between £200 and £800 plus VAT, depending on where you study it and how intensive the course is.

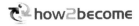

VTCT Level 3 in Nail Technology

As with the level 2 VTCT qualification, you can study Level 3 at local colleges and private colleges. This is normally a part-time course and you need to have Level 2 to enrol on the course.

This course covers the following:

- Manicure
- Pedicure
- Apply and maintain nails enhancements
- Design and apply nail art
- Enhance nails using electric files
- Display stock to promote sales in a salon
- Promote products and services to clients
- Maintain personal health and wellbeing
- Client care and communication
- Monitor and maintain health and safety practice in the salon.

The cost for this course is around £500 plus you will also have to provide funding for equipment as the course progresses.

Other Online Courses

There are many online courses advertised that say things like "You can learn to be a nail technician in just five days!" Unless the provider is offering one of the above qualifications it is unlikely that a prospective employer will accept your training with these providers.

Many of these courses are 'top-up' courses for already qualified nail technicians to enable them to learn a new skill or master a new technique. When you are a qualified nail technician you will need to do these types of courses too, in

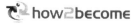

order to stay on top of your profession.

So as you can see, there are a lot of routes into becoming a nail technician, but before you choose your route I suggest you search for your course with care and only enrol on a course if it:

a) Meets your need

b) Meets your budget

c) Leads to a recognised qualification.

Habia, the government appointed sector skills body and industry authority for hair, beauty, nails, spa therapy, barbering and African type hair, has provided a guide to minimum skills that need to be taught to gain Level 2 and Level 3 qualifications as a nail technician which you can refer to when deciding if a course you have seen is suitable for you.

PRODUCT TRAINING

You can, also train to be a nail technician with one of the leading nail care product manufacturers like Opi, Jessica Nails and Bio Sculpture.

This will enable you to work as a nail technician, but won't guarantee you a job in a salon. Most salons will expect one of the more formal, recognised qualifications listed above. However, many work-from-home nail technicians have got by just fine with their product training.

Opi
To find an Opi training centre near you, do a search for Opi Training Centre and your region and you should see a list of salons and beauty institutes who offer Opi accredited training.

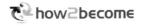

There are a wide range of Opi courses available from foundation courses, to manicure courses to advanced courses. These courses are quite short and you do come away with an Opi certificate.

The costs of these courses range from £1200 to £2000 but do include a full Opi kit to enable you to start work the moment you complete your course.

Opi also provides professional product training to qualified nail technicians. You need to be registered on the Opi site to gain access to the details of these courses.

Jessica Nails
This company does provide training but it is not very clear where you can train or how much it will cost. They require you to contact them directly to discuss your training requirements.

http://www.jessica-nails.co.uk/salon/

Bio-Sculpture
Bio-Sculpture offers a range of courses all over the country to train people as nail technicians.

Their basic manicure training (one day) covers all the important aspects of the formal qualifications including: anatomy, hand and nail diseases, hygiene and salon ethics, shaping and filing nails, manicures and hand massage and varnishes.

The company also offers courses on pedicures, gel training, gel extensions and nail art. You can find information on their courses here:

http://www.biosculpturegel.co.uk/

You will need to purchase the correct kit for your course as well as pay for the course itself, but as with Opi, this means

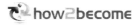

you can start to work to earn back your course fees as soon as you've completed your training. The course fee for the basic manicure training, including your kit comes to around £600.

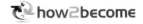

CHAPTER FIVE

CAREERS AS A NAIL TECHNICIAN

Once you have qualified as a nail technician you have a wide range of career options. You can choose to work in either an employed or self-employed capacity, full or part-time; it is an incredibly versatile career option.

Most people start out by working in a salon or nail bar, but you could just as easily start-up your own business.

Let's take a look at each career option in a bit more detail.

WORK IN A SALON

I say salon, but this could equally be a nail bar, in a hairdressing salon, a health club, a hotel spa, in a holiday resort or on a cruise ship. There is a huge demand for nail technicians in a wide variety of locations.

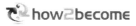

In a salon, or similar location, a nail technician will usually be expected to perform the following tasks:

- Present a neat, professional appearance at all times
- Wear a salon approved beauty technician tunic or uniform (you usually have to purchase this yourself)
- Make appointments for clients
- Keep client records
- Keep their work area clean and tidy
- Be responsible for the sterilisation of their equipment
- Be responsible for the stock levels of their equipment: varnishes, 3D designs, paints, lotions, creams, adhesives, fixatives, gel overlays, cuticle sticks, files etc.
- Carry out a wide range of manicures and pedicures as required by the salon.
- Keep themselves up to date with the latest in nail technology, designs and fashions by reading industry magazines such as Scratch, Professional Beauty and Vitality, and taking further courses as offered by Opi, Jessica Nails and Bio Sculpture.

In a salon, you will normally be expected to work around 37 hours a week full-time, and any number of hours part-time, depending upon your circumstances, your needs and the needs of the salon. Many of these hours will be unsocial – either evenings or weekends.

You can find jobs as a nail technician in a salon by checking in your local paper or by visiting the following job sites:

http://www.hair2beautyjobsource.com

http://www.indeed.co.uk/Nail-Technician-jobs

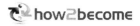

http://www.simplyhired.co.uk/

http://www.jobisjob.co.uk/

http://www.gumtree.com/

http://www.nailtechnicianjobs.org.uk/

To look for nail technician jobs abroad as well as in the UK check out:

http://www.leisurejobs.com/

To find a job on a cruise ship you need to visit the following sites:

http://www.onespaworld.com/

http://www.cruisejob1.com/

OWNER OF A NAIL BAR/SALON

After working in a salon for a few years many nail technicians go on to own their own nail bar or salon. However, you don't actually have to be a qualified nail technician to own a nail bar; you just need to ensure that your employees are skilled and experienced.

You can either buy an existing nail business or start one up from scratch. If you are looking to buy an existing business you can find them in your local commercial estate agents or on business for sale sites like Daltons and UK Businesses for Sale.

http://www.daltonsbusiness.com/

http://uk.businessesforsale.com/uk/

If you wish to convert an existing business into a nail salon, you must ensure it has A1 status.

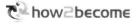

Whatever route you choose, you need to decide early on exactly what type of nail business you will operate. Will you run a walk-in nail bar offering mainly quick manicures or will you open a full nail salon offering a full range of treatments?

You also need to work out the minimum number of staff you need to employ to run an efficient business and where you will set up in business.

You will also need to undergo some sort of management training as you will now be responsible for the entire salon. This means you are responsible for the accounts, the insurance and in some towns, obtaining the licence needed to operate the salon. You will also need to be a skilled manager to manage your staff and grow your business. It is hard work, but can be tremendously rewarding. You can take management courses at most local colleges, online with the Open University or via specialist salon management courses like this one by Santi.

http://www.santi-santi.com/programmes.html

You need to decide on your budget and how you are going to fund this business. Estimates from people who have opened their own salons put the start up costs at between £20,000 and £50,000, with rents for salons at around £60,000 to £120,000 per year. Opening a salon is not a decision to take lightly!

BUSINESS PLANS

Setting up a business, whether it is opening a nail bar, working from home or as a mobile nail technician, will require capital. This means you need enough savings to buy all your equipment and products and cover your cost of living (if necessary) whilst building a client base. If you haven't

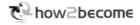

enough savings, then you will need to borrow the money in which case you will certainly need a business plan.

A business plan explains to banks what you hope to achieve in your business, how and when.

It consists of the following sections:

- **Executive Summary** (What your business does, where the market opportunity is, who you expect your clients to be, when you expect to make a profit). The summary basically sums up everything you've written in the business plan, which is why it makes sense to write this section last.

- **The Business Opportunity** – Why you are setting up your business.

- **Your Marketing Strategy** – How you are going to attract your clients, how you are going to set your rates, what rates you will charge etc.

- **Your Skills** – (and in the case of a partnership or limited company – the skills of any staff you will or need to recruit.)

- **Your Place of Operations** – Where you will be based, cost of any equipment needed etc.

- **Financial Forecasts** – How well you expect to do based on your experience of the industry and other similar nail bars you have researched.

You can find a guide to producing a business plan here: http://www.businesslink.gov.uk/

Business Link has comprehensive advice, articles and videos on setting up your own business.

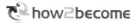

WORKING FROM HOME

"I am self employed, home based," said Isabella when we asked her where she works. She continued: *"I am disabled and can't walk very well. My husband has helped me set up a room at home with everything I need."*

Many nail technicians, once qualified, choose to set themselves up in business by working from home. There are many advantages to this:

- No commute
- No salon rent costs
- No staff costs
- You get to be your own boss
- You get to choose when you work

However, before setting up your business from home, consider whether there is demand for nail treatments in the area that you live and whether there is any local competition.

You may come to the conclusion that offering the services and flexibility associated with a mobile nail technician may be a better option for you in the first instance. Once you have established yourself within your local area, clients may be more willing to travel to your home. There is no right or wrong answer but I would advise doing some research first on your target market to help you decide the best route to take. We will cover your target market later in the book.

If you choose to work from home as a nail technician you must first of all discover whether you need a licence to promote your nail technician business from your local council. You then need to sort out a professional workspace in your home that you will use as your treatment room.

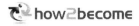

This room needs to be welcoming and professional looking. You will need suitable furniture and equipment so that your clients feel comfortable and get as much of a 'salon' experience as they can. You will also need strong, lockable cupboards for your chemicals and equipment as well as a sterilizer unit.

You might find it handy to have a separate telephone line for your business so that you can keep work and personal calls separate.

You will need to keep your own appointments and your own accounting records. You will have to notify HMRC that you have set up in business as a sole trader – more on that below.

You will have to purchase insurance for your business and you will also be responsible for your own marketing.

MOBILE WORKING

As an alternative to working from your own home, many nail technicians set up a mobile nail technician service, visiting clients in their own homes.

There are many advantages to this method of working:

- Home life and working life are kept separate
- It gets you out of the house
- You choose your hours of work
- You are your own boss

However, you will need a suitable car to transport all your equipment and you will need suitable, strong containers for your chemicals and equipment. You will also need to factor petrol costs into your expenses and you will still need to purchase insurance, do your accounting and your own

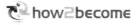

marketing. As with working from home, depending on where you live, you might also need to obtain a licence from your local council.

TEACHING/DEMONSTRATING AT COLLEGES/NAIL PRODUCT COMPANIES

After working as a nail technician for several years, many nail technicians go on to teach others how to become a nail technician and gain work at local colleges, nail institutes like Essential Nails, The Nail Company or Next Step Beauty or with nail product companies like Opi, Bio Sculpture and Jessica Nails.

You can find such vacancies by searching the local paper in the case of college jobs or online. If you have identified companies that you might like to work for, contact them directly regarding career opportunities.

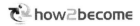

CHAPTER SIX

WHAT SERVICES SHOULD YOU OFFER IF SETTING UP ON YOUR OWN?

"These days I only do the Bio Sculpture gel system nails. It is more natural looking and kinder to your nails. I find the acrylic too fake looking and there is a lot of buffing involved with acrylic which can damage the nails," said Emma.

"I generally do manicures, pedicures, and gels," answered Danielle who works in a salon.

Whereas Isabella, who like Emma works from home, said she offers: *"Silk and acrylic nail extensions and wraps, nail art, Shellac & Gelish gel polish, manicure and pedicure."*

If you are thinking of setting up on your own as a nail technician, either from home or mobile, then you need to work out what

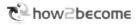

services you are going to offer and how you are going to work. Working for yourself is tremendously rewarding but is also a lot of hard work, especially in the beginning. To make your business work you need to do the following:

1. Research Your Market
2. Target Your Clients
3. Decide what nail treatments you would like to offer
4. Decide what products you would like to use
5. Consider Your Competition
6. Keep Up-to-date

RESEARCH YOUR MARKET

This is crucial to the success or failure of your business. You need to know who is using the services of a nail technician in your area and how you are going to attract them.

If there are no nail technicians in your local area you need to consider why:

- Is there any demand for nail technicians in this area?

- Have any nail technician businesses started up here in the past?

If you think there is demand that no-one is satisfying, this could be a good place to set up your business.

If you are based from home or mobile, you can target several areas with your marketing. Before you do this, you need to work out what people are currently paying and what services they are using. This will help you decide what services to offer and what to charge. I suggest talking to as many people as possible – friends, family, friends of friends, work

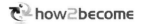

colleagues, etc. In other words, everyone you can think of in your network that may have an opinion on nail treatments! You can start to collate the information to show popular nail treatments, the latest and up and coming nail trends and the costs of such treatments.

TARGET YOUR CLIENTS

Who do you want as clients? You might think you want every possible client you can get, but do you? Do you want a high turnover of quick manicure treatments and file and paints or do you want clients who want a luxury manicure or pedicure, extensions and airbrush designs?

Think about what type of work you would prefer to do and target accordingly. If you are happy for lots of quick jobs, target your marketing to people who are likely to want this. If, on the other hand, you would rather concentrate on luxury treatments, then you will need to work out how to reach those customers instead.

DECIDE WHAT TREATMENTS YOU WOULD LIKE TO OFFER

Now draw up your list of treatments bearing in mind three key questions:

1. Is this treatment in demand?
2. Am I qualified to provide this treatment professionally and skilfully to meet my clients' expectations?
3. Do I want to provide this treatment – will I enjoy it or not?

If the answer to any of these questions is no, then delete that treatment from your list.

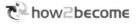

To help you draw up your list of treatments, use our Treatment Matrix Worksheet to help you match your skills and experience against the treatments that clients' want.

Treatment	Qualified/ Skills/ Experience	Local Demand Yes/No	Do I want to offer this treatment?
Nail art	Yes	No	No
Nail extensions	Yes	Yes	Yes
Manicures – basic	Yes	Yes	Yes
Manicures – luxury	Yes	Unknown	Yes
French manicure	Yes	Yes	Yes
Japanese manicure	No	Unknown	Not yet
Hot Oil Manicures	Yes	Unknown	Yes
Paraffin Dips	Yes	Unknown	Yes
Pedicures – basic	Yes	Yes	Yes
Pedicures – luxury	Yes	Unknown	Yes
Gel wraps	No	Yes	Possibly - need training
Acrylic extensions	Yes	Yes	Yes
Nail repair	Yes	Yes	Yes

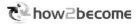

Remember, this list is not set in stone; you can add and delete treatments as your business matures. You may decide that you would like to offer a large selection of treatments or specialise in just a few.

DECIDE WHAT PRODUCTS YOU WOULD LIKE TO USE

This is one of the best aspects of being your own boss; you get to decide what products to use!

But make sure you consider the following points before making a decision on products:

1. Is there a particular product that you are already trained in using or would you like to take this opportunity to choose another well-known and respected brand? If you trained with Opi or Bio-Sculpture, it makes sense to continue to use those products as you will have them in your kit.

2. Look at your target market – what types of products will your potential clients' like?

3. If you choose a professional product – how easy will it be to buy stock and will there be a minimum order requirement?

4. Will you offer a range of products?

Do your research and make sure you are fully up to date on the latest trends and product ranges on the market. Some well respected big names in the nail industry include Opi, Bio-Sculpture and Jessica Nails and these are popular with ladies who have their nails done on a regular basis. These are the brands they see in salons and the brands they trust. Many leading brands such as Opi, Bio-Sculpture and Jessica Nails will offer training programmes to cover their products and treatments.

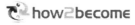

- Bio-Sculpture
  http://biosculpturegel.co.uk/content.aspx?ContentID=6

- Jessica Nails
  http://www.jessica-nails.co.uk/salon/

- Opi
  http://pro.opi.com/logon.aspx

A great place to sample products and learn about up and coming new trends is by attending Trade Shows, which are held in various cities throughout the country. Suppliers often give special discounts for introductory offers and it is also a good opportunity to network with other nail technicians and beauty therapists.

CONSIDER YOUR COMPETITION

This is crucial; you need to give your potential clients a reason to come to you and not to go to a salon or other mobile or home-based technician. So you need to find out as much as you can about your competition. You might need to go undercover here and pose as a client to find out what services your competitors are offering; what products they use and what they charge. You should also carry out some online research, as many beauty and nail salons will have a website showing their list of treatments, the brand of products used and pricing structure.

Armed with this information you can set your own prices and determine your own services. Aim to offer something different; be it better quality products, a wider or narrower range of services and appropriate prices.

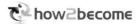

KEEP UP-TO-DATE

Once you have got your business up and running you cannot afford to rest on your laurels. You need to ensure you can continue to meet the needs of your clients. This means you will need to read nail technician magazines such as Scratch, Professional Beauty and Vitality and take further professional development courses such as ones held by Opi, Jessica Nails and Bio Sculpture.

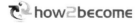

CHAPTER SEVEN

SETTING UP AT HOME OR YOUR MOBILE NAIL TECHNICIAN BUSINESS

There are many reasons for starting up your own nail technician business, either based at home or as a mobile service. The main reasons people choose to set up on their own are:

- **Flexibility** – you choose when and where you work and what hours you work. And it is easier to take time off and reschedule appointments if a family commitment means you are needed elsewhere.

- **You are Your Own Boss** – you choose your wages, your holidays, your uniform and the services you offer.

- **A Sense of Freedom** – people like to work for themselves; it can be very liberating.

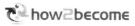

HOW TO SET UP IN BUSINESS IN THE UK

First of all you need to decide if you're going to be a sole-trader, a partnership or a limited company.

There is more to this than just the choice of name. The type of business you choose to set up has implications for accounting, tax, National Insurance, shares of profits and liabilities for debts.

SOLE TRADER

A sole trader is the easiest of all structures. You work for and by yourself. You alone are entitled to the profits and you alone are responsible for the debts. If you are renting a room in a salon, you are a sole trader.

There is a guide to the advantages of setting up a sole trader and the steps involved in doing so here: http://businesslink.gov.uk/static/html/layer-978.html

To set up as a sole trader you simply need to register your new business with the HMRC. http://hmrc.gov.uk/selfemployed/

As a sole trader you receive all profits and pay all tax on profits. You need to pay tax (once a year) and pay National Insurance Contributions Class 2 and Class 4.

You will need to complete a tax return at the end of the tax year and pay tax on your earnings in the previous tax year. When you pay your tax you will also need to pay your Class 4 National Insurance Contributions. You will pay Class 2 NI contributions every quarter.

The HMRC has lots of useful courses and videos on becoming self-employed that you might find useful, explaining accounts, keeping records, legal issues, paying Class 2 and Class 4

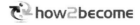

National Insurance Contributions etc. As a business owner you own all the business equipment but are also solely liable for all the business' debts. You may use a business name other than your own name for your business but your real name as owner, must be listed on all stationery, business cards, documents and business emails.

- As a sole trader you do not need to prepare complicated accounts or balance sheets.

- There are no set-up costs in becoming a Sole Trader.

PARTNERSHIP

If you are starting out in business as a partnership, you and your partner(s) are legally responsible for the debts of the business and also share the profits of the business in proportion to your partnership agreement.

You will need a solicitor to draw up a partnership agreement. You can find advice on setting up in business as a partnership here:

http://www.businesslink.gov.uk/

You will still pay tax once a year and both Class 2 and Class 4 National Insurance Contributions.

LIMITED LIABILITY PARTNERSHIP (LLP)

This structure offers partnerships a limit to the amount of debt they, as partners, are liable for. There is advice on how to set up a limited liability partnership (LLP) here: http://www.businesslink.gov.uk/

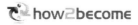

LIMITED COMPANY

A Limited Company means that as owner, your liability for debts is limited to what you have invested in the company.

If you wish to set up your business as a limited company then this is a lot more involved than setting up as a sole trader or partnership. A limited company is a legal entity. This means that the company is responsible for its debts and the company, not you, makes the profit and pays the taxes. The company then pays you a wage or salary or bonus and you will pay tax on that.

Your Limited Company needs to be incorporated with Companies House. You will need a Memorandum of Association and an Articles of Association and to fill in lots of forms!

You can buy a 'off the shelf' company and just change the name with Companies House and this is a quicker way of setting up a limited company. Here are a few of the better known companies offering this service:

http://www.companyregistration.uk-plc.net

http://www.ltd-companies.co.uk/

http://www.paramountformations.com

You must also have properly prepared accounts and balance sheets each year and file your accounts with Companies House.

At the moment the majority of nail technicians in the UK are sole-traders, which isn't that surprising.

It is easy to set-up as a sole trader and is free!

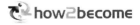

TO SET UP AS A SOLE TRADER

You need to notify Her Majesty's Revenue and Customs (HMRC) within 100 days of starting up in business, that you have started a business as a sole-trader, if you fail to do this, you can get fined. To register with HMRC you need to either visit www.businesslink.gov.uk/taxhelp or call the Newly Self-Employed Helpline on 0845 915 4515.

If you are unsure which business model is right for you, check out the huge range of training videos and e-learning modules available for free online by Business Link: http://businesslink.gov.uk/

Most nail technicians I spoke to also strongly recommend attending a newly self-employed course run by HMRC, you can find details of them here, as well as free booklets and other advice on starting your own business: http://hmrc.gov.uk/

ACCOUNTS AND RECORDS

No matter what structure you choose for your business, you will need to keep some basic financial records.

If you are a sole-trader or a partnership, a simple spreadsheet program or cash book will suffice. Keep an accurate record of your incomings and expenses and all receipts relevant to your business and use these to help you complete your tax return.

And when it comes to keeping records, there are several applications you can download to keep track of your business receipts and expenses.

Some highly recommended ones used by nail technicians working from home are:

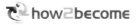

- NCH Software http://www.nchsoftware.com/
- QuickBooks http://www.intuit.co.uk/

Accurate records will also be handy when it comes to business banking or asking for a business loan.

If you are a limited liability partnership or limited company, you will need an accountant to prepare your accounts for you. Business bank managers will expect to see accounts for limited companies.

WHAT'S IN A NAME?

Before you register your business you need to think of a name for it. It has to be something that sounds professional and that conveys the correct image for your nail technician business and the clients you wish to attract.

Bitty Nails doesn't sound very attractive! Well, I wouldn't want to go there! And if you name happens to be Boots, you cannot use that as the name for your business as Boots the Chemist will object!

First of all, take a look at some other nail technician businesses to get an idea for the kind of names they use. Look at existing businesses in your local area and search for nail technicians online to see what types of business names they are using.

You want a name that is professional, but not one that can be easily mistaken for another nail technician; your clients could end up going to your competitor instead!

Before deciding on which name to use for your business, remember that as a Sole Trader your business name does not have to be your name.

Think about your target audience and the typical internet

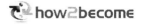

search a potential client might use to find a nail technician in your area. Knowing what people are searching for will help you to find the right name for your business and help your potential clients find you.

It is a good idea to research a domain name with your location e.g. Nail Technician Manchester or Nail Technician Buckinghamshire. Make sure that your domain name starts with the key phrases that is being searched and does not include any dashes. Note that potential clients in the UK are sub-consciously looking for a co.uk

Your domain name might look something like this:

www.nailartist.co.uk

www.nailartmanchester.co.uk

www.nailtech.co.uk

www.justnails.co.uk

I suggest doing an online search to see if anyone else is currently using that name or one like it.

As soon as you have decided on the perfect name for your business, you need to think about registering your domain name. You might not think this is essential for a nail technician, but you would be wrong!

Most of us search for everything on the internet these days, and people looking for a nail technician are no different. If you are going to attract all the clients you possibly can from your area you will need a website. And the first step in getting a website is getting a domain name.

So, check your domain name is available before deciding on which business name you are going to use.

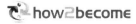

I suggest checking out the following sites to choose and register your domain name. Do this now and we'll talk about setting up your web site later. You don't want someone else stealing your name when you've spent so long coming up with it!

http://order.1and1.co.uk/ this site offers .co.uk domains from as little as £2.49 a year, and .com domains from £6.99 a year. It also offers web hosting.

http://123-reg.co.uk/ offers domain names, web hosting and a variety of web hosting accounts.

As well as registering the domain, you need to find a web host to host your site. Many of the above also offer web hosting, but look around to ensure you get the best hosting for you. You need a site with support (based in this country ideally), and that offers the facilities you are looking for in the site, such as email accounts for your business and an easy way to update the site and a low period of downtime.

Try to avoid free hosting if possible as the adverts you get on the site will detract from the site and make it look less professional.

http://www.fastvision.com/ This site offers a vast array of domain extensions from .co.uk at £2.99 a year, but also .org, .net, uk.com and many, many more.

Many web designers these days advise their clients to buy as many variations on their domain name as possible and to at least buy the .com, .co.uk and .biz extensions. This is to prevent people setting up an account with the same name as yours but with a different extension on which they put up unsavoury material. Such sites can seriously affect your site and these people will only take them down if you buy the domain from them; normally at a very inflated price.

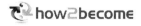

GETTING ADVICE ON SETTING UP YOUR BUSINESS

Before you start up your own business, you need to get as much advice as you can from people who can help you.

Try talking with other nail technicians at http://salongeek.com/ especially those who have set up their own business to get their industry specific advice.

The nail technicians I spoke to recommend the following sources of business advice:

Business Link
Business Link has a great website with videos, tutorials and print outs to help you get your business up and running: http://www.businesslink.gov.uk/

HMRC
Attending a Becoming Self-Employed Course by the HMRC is also highly recommended, plus they have some booklets for the newly self-employed too: http://www.hmrc.gov.uk/

Start-ups.co.uk
A site aimed at people starting up their own business. http://www.startups.co.uk/

Small business.co.uk
A site for small businesses, which has articles on management, staff, law, marketing, accounting etc. http://smallbusiness.co.uk/

You should also consider talking to your bank about setting up a business bank account and getting their help and support for your business. Many banks offer free or reduced rate business banking for the first few months.

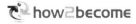

Alternatively you could talk to an accountant about your plans. And speaking of banks and accountants, you need to think about money.

HOW MUCH MONEY WILL YOU NEED TO INVEST?

"My running cost for last year was £6562.00. But this can change from year to year depending on how busy I have been," said Emma, who runs her business from home.

Isabella also works from home, but she responded that: *"My running costs are on average about 12k per year, my gross for this year is 21k and I work on my own."*

This is a tough one to answer and it depends on what you already have and whether you are working from home or mobile.

You should already have your nail kit and most varnishes etc. To work for yourself you will also need a full range of varnishes, polishes, adhesives, fixatives, cleaning and sterilizing equipment, cuticle sticks, emery boards etc.

Emma did a quick calculation of the cost of equipment needed and she came up with the following:

1.	Cuticle nippers	£3.49
2.	Gel lamp	£59.00
3.	Box of tips	£12.49
4.	Stork scissors	£2.95
5.	Cuticle pusher	£2.95
6.	Pack of nail files 80 to 180 Grit	£2.50
7.	Gel Brush	£3.95
8.	Barbiside solution	£5.99

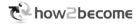

9.	Nail glue	£7.95
10.	Top coat	£9.95
11.	Tip Cutters	£6.00
12.	Table protector paper roll	£3.95
13.	Lint free wipes	£6.95
14.	A towel as cheap as	£3.00
15.	Sanitizer	£4.00
16.	Nail varnish remover	£4.00
17.	Bio sculpture Clear gel 10ml	£32.00
18.	Each 4ml pot of Bio Sculpture Colour Gel (Recommended 5 colours to start with)	£16.50

Apart from the Bio Sculpture products you can pick up all the other stock from anywhere. Look around for the cheapest. I took these prices out of a magazine I had called Salonserve. So these prices are a guide only. Also this does not include VAT.

Total £253.62

Whereas, Danielle, who works in a salon confirmed that it cost her around £500 to purchase her nail kit.

As you can see, the costs involved can vary considerably.

If you are working from home you need to purchase a salon chair and suitable storage furniture for your equipment as well as a work table and a UV lamp.

If you are mobile, you need to purchase suitable storage containers to hold your equipment and chemicals as you move around.

However, for most nail technicians you can get started in business for a few thousand pounds.

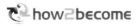

Use your qualified status to buy your products and equipment at health and beauty wholesalers and use your contacts in the industry and SalonGeek to find the best deals on salon furniture.

EQUIPMENT AND PRODUCTS NEEDED

As a minimum you will need to have the following:

- A salon chair
- A worktable
- A light
- A UV lamp
- A range of emery boards
- Orange cuticle sticks
- Hoof stick
- Foot file
- Nail files
- Nail buffers
- Nail buffing cream
- Nail scissors
- Cuticle Tip tool
- Face masks
- Tunic
- Cutting blade (for acrylic nails)
- Picker (for gemstones)
- Foam wipes
- Cotton pieces
- Finger soakers
- Nail art tip stand

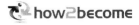

- A range of varnishes
- Varnish remover
- Cuticle oil
- Cuticle cream
- Spatulas
- Hand lotions
- Base coats
- Top coats
- Dappen dish (if applying extensions, tips, acrylic nails etc)
- Nail dryer
- Nail brushes (a variety)
- Disinfecting Jars
- Pedicure bowls/foot spas
- Pedicure wash
- Pedicure scrubs
- Hard skin removers (electric)
- Pedicure lotions
- Pedicure masks
- Manicure bowl
- Manicure masks
- Nail Tips
- Gemstones
- Nail wraps
- Gel overlays

You will also need to pay for marketing materials: leaflets, posters, adverts as well as your website.

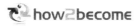

HOW MANY HOURS WILL YOU NEED TO PUT INTO YOUR BUSINESS

This is entirely up to you, but you will have to put more hours in at the beginning than at any other time. So even if you intend to only work part-time, you will find that you need to work many more hours at first to get your business off the ground.

You will need to leaflet drop areas to get your name out there which can take some time. Plus you will need to work on your site and come up with ways to attract as many clients as possible, such as offering an opening week special – which you will need to get into the local press so people know it is happening.

Even when your business is up and running you will need to spend on average ten hours a week on maintaining your business: doing your record keeping, accounts, admin and most importantly marketing your business.

DOWNSIDE OF BEING SELF-EMPLOYED

While there are lots of advantages to being self-employed, there are, it has to be said, some disadvantages too.

- **Low Earnings** – At first you have to put every penny into building your business and it can be a while before you earn anything which can put people off.

- **Loneliness** – Many people find it lonely working on their own, so if you are someone who always needs to be with other people, then this is probably not the right option for you.

- **Unpaid Holidays** – When you take holidays as a

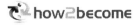

self-employed person you lose money. And unless you notify your clients well in advance and have built up good client relationships, you can lose your clients whilst on holiday and they might not come back.

- **No Sick Pay** – Likewise, if you are ill you lose your earnings that day and could lose your client. For these two reasons alone you must work hard to build not only good, but great client relationships so that your clients won't mind if you are ill or go on holiday.

- **Motivation** – You have to motivate yourself to get to work every day – no-one else is going to do it! It can be hard to keep motivated day after day.

You can get around most of these by talking to other nail technicians and realising that you are not alone. This is where sites such as SalonGeek come in handy.

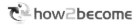

CHAPTER EIGHT

FINANCIAL AWARENESS AND GUIDANCE

WHAT WILL YOUR EARNING POTENTIAL BE?

In a salon in the UK you can earn between £12,000 and £25,000 per annum. As a self-employed nail technician, however, you are in charge of setting your own rates and thus you are, to a certain extent, responsible for how much you earn.

A key factor in how much you earn is how much you charge for your services.

SETTING COMPETITIVE RATES

Isabella told us how she sets her rates: *"I tend to look at my competition, my level of experience and training. I am not the cheapest around my area, but I do very well."*

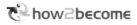

"I pop in to 3 local beauty salons," said Emma, *"and pick up a price list. I then mark my prices somewhere in between."*

You cannot charge as much as a salon as you are not offering a salon experience, so your rates will need to be discounted compared to those in salons.

You will need to work out what rates are charged in salons or by other self-employed or mobile technicians for their treatments and then set your own competitive rates. You don't want to be the cheapest as that will put off several of the better-off clients who would be likely to want a luxury manicure or pedicure, as they will think you are not skilled. Plus you need to make a profit!

From talking to other technicians, here is a general guide as to the rates being charged for treatments:

File and Paint	£6 – £15
Basic Manicure	£20 – £30
Basic Pedicure	£25 – £40
French Manicure	£4 – £12
	(charged in addition to basic manicure)
Luxury Manicures	£20 – £40
Luxury Pedicure	£30 – £45
Gel/Acrylic Nails	£30 – 35 (full set)
Extension Removal	£15 – £30
Nail Repair	£2.50 – £5.00 per nail
Nail Art	£.0.50 – £2.50 per nail

Talk to other technicians on SalonGeek to find out what they are doing and how they set their rates and visit the websites of several nail technicians to get an idea for how they price their services.

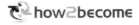

HOW TO MAXIMISE YOUR INCOME

The best way to maximise your income is to offer additional services such as:

- Mini manicures and pedicures,
- Nail parties (incredibly popular with girls aged 8 – 12)
- Wedding nails
- Luxury manicures and pedicures
- Selling nail care products

SELLING PRODUCTS TO MAKE A PROFIT

As a qualified nail technician you can purchase your nail varnishes, removers, boards, files, lotions etc at wholesale prices.

You can then sell these products onto your clients at retail prices to make a profit.

Customers do not like a hard sell, but they might be persuaded to purchase a lotion or varnish if you recommend it to them as a way of maintaining their manicure, nails etc.

KEEPING RECORDS

As a nail technician you need to keep two sets of records:

- Client records
- Financial records

CLIENT RECORDS

You need to keep track of your clients, who you've seen, what you did, what treatments they wanted etc, to make it

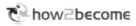

easier for you to give this client a personal service.

You also need to work out a system for making appointments and sending out reminders to clients so that you keep getting repeat business and thus more income.

Many nail technicians use appointment books and customer file cards for this, but you can, if you prefer, purchase software which not only manages your client records but your financial records too.

Three of the most popular salon software systems are:

http://www.i-salonsoftware.co.uk

http://www.studiotracker.co.uk/

http://www.phorest.com

FINANCIAL RECORDS

As a self-employed nail technician you are responsible for paying your own tax and National Insurance.

If you are a sole-trader you do not need to keep detailed accounts BUT you must keep a record of your incomings and expenses. You must also keep a copy of your invoices, payments received, bills, and receipts that relate to your business.

I suggest using software or an accounts book to record your incomings and expenses, which you should rule off and total month by month. Use one page for incomings and one for expenses. This makes it so much easier when it comes to doing your tax return.

List your expenses and give each one a number e.g. May1201, May1202 etc and write this number on the relevant receipt.

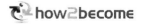

Keep your receipts in envelopes or clear plastic wallets for each calendar month.

If you prefer to use software for this, you can get free trials of accounting software on Google Apps and from most accounting software programs. Some of the most popular ones are:

- NCH Software http://www.nchsoftware.com/

- QuickBooks http://www.intuit.co.uk/

You will need all of this information to help you complete your tax return. You need to submit your tax return by either the 31st October of the tax year if you want the Inland Revenue to calculate your tax bill, or by 31st January, if you are going to calculate your tax bill yourself. You will then be told how much your tax bill will be and the dates on which you need to have paid it. It is normal for tax bills to be split into two instalments. If you fail to submit your tax return on time or fail to make a payment deadline, you will be fined.

You can either complete your tax return yourself, and it is quite easy to do, especially as the Inland Revenue provides lots of advice, or you can pay an accountant to do this for you.

You will also need to pay both Class 2 and Class 4 National Insurance Contributions. Class 2 are paid quarterly and Class 4 contributions are paid annually, at the same time as your tax bill.

There is more advice on accounting records, tax and National Insurance for the self-employed on the HMRC website here:

http://www.hmrc.gov.uk/

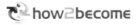

TAX AND LEGAL IMPLICATIONS

Tax Issues

As a self-employed nail technician, you will be able to claim some of your expenses as a tax deductible expense – not all your expenses are tax deductible!

You should always check with an accountant as the rules for what are and aren't tax deductible can change, but at the moment you can claim the following as tax deductible expenses:

- Rent (for your room in a salon)

- A proportion of the running costs of your vehicle (if providing a mobile service)

- Equipment purchases for the business (salon chair, UV lamp, steriliser etc)

- Products purchased for use in the business

- Insurance

- Pension Contributions

Legal Issues

You will also need to purchase indemnity insurance for your business to protect you should your clients suffer any injury whilst on your premises or under your care. The following companies offer suitable insurance for nail technicians:

The Beauty Guild http://www.beautyguild.com

http://www.salonsaver.co.uk/justfornails.htm

http://www.professionalbeauty.co.uk

http://www.abtinsurance.co.uk/

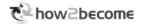

CHAPTER NINE
HOW TO ATTRACT CLIENTS

"I find that nail technicians do not usually pick up that many clients through advertising," said Emma. *"It is normally word of mouth, or client recommendations. I have been so lucky that I have kept the same clients for many years. But I have in the past advertised in the local newspapers, I have done school pamper evenings, and popped flyers into letterboxes."*

"I advertise in local ad magazines," said Isabella, *"but not newspapers as people save the ad magazines and throw away papers."*

When you set up in business by yourself, naturally you want to attract clients, someone to pay you to do what you are good at. However, before we get too carried away here, it is important to think about the clients you want to attract to make sure you only attract those clients and not clients who make you wish you'd never started up in business in the first

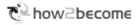

place. So to avoid making bad decisions and getting stuck in a terrible working relationship, here are some tips on what to look for in a client when you are targeting them.

WHAT TYPE OF CLIENT DO YOU WANT?

When you are thinking of your clients, who do you see coming through your door?

- How old are they?
- Where do they live?
- What job do they do?
- When will they visit you – evening, daytime, weekends?
- What services will they want?

Use your findings from this to work out who your clients are likely to be and work out how you can attract their attention.

Are your ideal clients stay-at-home mums? Think about targeting nurseries and schools.

Are they working women? Target office buildings and cafes near office blocks with your marketing material?

Do they live in your local area? Target the local shops to see if they will carry cards or leaflets advertising your services.

We work best with people who are like us. That is just a fact of life. So think about where you shop, where you spend your leisure time, where you live and chances are that this is where you will find your ideal client.

Remember, it takes time to build up a new business. Most self-employed nail technicians I spoke to said it takes on average six months to get the business working properly. So here are some ideas on how to get your clients coming in.

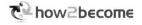

SHOW YOUR NAILS TO THE WORLD

This is such a simple idea but one that really works. Simply do your nails so that they look fantastic and go out and about. When people compliment you on your nails, tell them you did them yourself and you are a nail technician. Have a handy supply of business cards or postcards with your details on and a discount voucher.

THINK OUTSIDE THE BOX

Visit the local retirement homes to see if any of the residents there would like their nails doing – this way you get to make one trip for hopefully, a lot of clients.

Visit local hotels and ask if you can leave your leaflets/postcards in their reception or even have them included in the 'in-room' packs that hotels make up for their guests.

Contact large corporate organisations to see if you can offer nail technician services at lunchtime or directly after work to their employees.

Visit local weight-loss groups and advertise your services there – either in person or via leaflets/postcards.

Approach hairdressing salons and see if you can link up to provide nail treatments whilst clients are having their hair done.

GIVE THEM A REASON TO COME TO YOU

Give all your customers a discount for their first few visits. Make sure all your marketing material includes a discount voucher or code. Put discount codes on your website and Facebook pages. But not only that, make sure you are

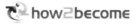

offering something no-other nail technician is: make a big deal of your nail art skills, your manicure skills or your skills with gels. Give your clients as many reasons as possible to try your services.

OFFER THEM A GUARANTEE

Nothing reassures customers more than a guarantee that they won't be risking their money. Make your guarantee simple, achievable and measurable. If, for example, you are offering nail extensions your guarantee could be something like "no lifting guaranteed for two weeks." Make sure, however, that whatever guarantee you make you can keep!

REWARD LOYALTY

Give your customers a loyalty card with discounts or with points that they can collect to earn a free mini-manicure or other service. This will encourage them to keep coming back.

MARKET!

Get the word out about your business in every way you possibly can. This is something you don't just do when you are starting your business, but throughout the life of your business. If you don't market, don't advertise your services, how will anyone know to come to you?

MAKE THE MOST OF YOUR USP

Your USP is your Unique Selling Point and you will have one; everyone does. It could be that you are the only nail technician in your area offering gel overlays, or airbrush

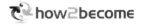

designs. It could be that you're young or that you're middle aged and experienced. It could be that you are a Goth or a Science-fiction fan.

Look at the other nail technicians in business in your town and work out your unique selling point and make sure you make the most of it in your marketing materials and on your website.

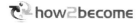

CHAPTER TEN

MARKETING YOUR BUSINESS

There are two potential strategies you can take when it comes to marketing: a mass blast or a targeted approach. A mass blast is easier to do, but is expensive and is not very effective. With a mass blast approach you would post your postcards, leaflets or brochures through as many doors as you can, or leave them in every waiting room you find. But before you consider this approach, think about it; how many of the people receiving these leaflets will be interested in your services?

If, however, you use a targeted marketing approach, sending your details only to clients who are likely to need your services and are able to pay for your services, not only will your marketing costs be lower, but your chances of success will be higher.

So the first step in drawing up your marketing plan and

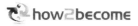

starting to market your business is to decide what type of clients you want to work with and drawing their attention to your business.

The key to marketing your business, however, is that you must start before you are ready to start work. You need to drum up business in order for you to have any business to do!

And you cannot stop marketing your business even when you have got some clients. You must still put aside some time each week for marketing activities

But what exactly are you marketing and how should you go about it?

ESTABLISHING YOUR BUSINESS IDENTITY

This is vital. You need to work out and spell out what makes your nail technician business different from others in your area. You need to come up with your Unique Selling Point or USP.

You need to work on your skills and services list and work out a way to present all the services you can offer your potential clients.

This is where your Business Name and Logo also come into play. A professional name and a good logo work together to make your business look professional; it inspires trust in prospective clients.

Do your research; download articles, take a look at several other nail technician websites to see how they set themselves apart and how they market their services and then see what you can come up with for your site.

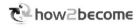

Don't copy anything directly from these sites as you will just look like everyone else and the only way you can compete with these other nail technicians will be on price. Besides which, copying from websites is in fact plagiarism and can be punished by your Internet Service Provider removing your website!

BRANDING YOUR BUSINESS

Logo

A logo instantly makes a business look more professional. You can either design your own logo or have one professionally designed for you. Do keep your logo and brand crisp and professional looking. You can hire logo designers at freelance work sites or have them designed for you online for as little as £50.

Think carefully about colours as this will also affect the colour scheme for your website and your professional stationery.

Most logo designers will ask you about your business and the clients you want to attract during their initial consultation to design your logo. Also, most will come up with a choice of at least three logos for you to choose from and offer free revisions.

Setting up your Website

By now you should have already bought your domain name for your nail technician business. If not, look back to Chapter 7 and do it now!

Now you need to design your website and fill it full of content. You can either do this yourself using WYSIWYG (What You See is what you Get) editors available on some ISPS or using HTML or software like DreamWeaver or WordPress.

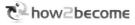

A fabulous website I came across recently is http://wix.com. You can choose from a selection of templates to design your own website or Facebook page and then simply download photos and insert content yourself. This is a really simple way to create your own website and it is relatively cheap to run their premium package, which includes your own domain name, search engine optimisation tools and more.

If you'd rather not get involved in creating your own site then you can hire a freelancer via freelancing websites such as Elance, Guru, ODesk or VWorker, or ask around in the SalonGeek forum for advice and recommendations to hire someone else to design your website for you.

Your website must look professional. No spelling mistakes, no typos, no bad links, no inappropriate music or flashy graphics. It must impress.

As an absolute minimum your Website needs the following pages:

Home Page: This is the first page a potential client looks at when they type in your web address. This is your landing page and you have about 10 to 15 seconds to make a positive impression! This page is your main sales page. So make it look good! Use photos, colours and fonts to create a warm, yet professional salon experience on your home page.

Photos: You are selling a beauty service, and people want to see examples of your work. So put up photos of your work on line, either on the home page or in a portfolio section so that clients can see what you do.

Services Page: List the services you offer and your fees. Many nail technicians also list the brand of products they use here, to reassure potential clients that they only use the best professional brands such as Jessica Nail, Bio Sculpture or Opi.

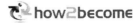

About Page: This is where you sing your own praises. List your experiences, your qualifications, jobs you have done, anything to set you apart from other nail technicians and make the client consider choosing you to do their nails. Again include photos of your work if possible.

FAQ Page: Come up with questions a client might have about manicures, pedicures, extensions, gel overlays etc and answer them. This reassures clients that you know what you are talking about!

Contact Page: Provide at least a phone number and a contact form, so people can contact you via email. Don't just put your email address up on the site or you will be inundated with spam!

Clients/Testimonials Page: Full of positive client testimonials. I can't stress enough the importance of client testimonials. The majority of us are influenced by testimonials and potential clients will be no different.

Optional Pages

Blog: You can write a blog on news that is relevant to the nail technician industry or to your clients.

Video: This is a great way of introducing yourself to potential clients and explaining the services you can offer. Video is becoming more and more popular on websites these days and a YouTube video with a link back to your website is great for moving your website up the rankings in Google. Higher page rankings mean that a potential client is more likely to come across your website when they are looking for a nail technician.

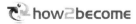

GETTING TRAFFIC TO YOUR WEBSITE

First of all, check your site looks good on all browsers. If you have hired a web designer, ensure they also do this for you. Browsershots enables you to do this for free. http://browsershots.org/

Once you're happy that your site looks good no matter which browser is used, you need to list your site so it will start to show up in Search Results.

Now get your site listed at Google, http://www.google.com/submityourcontent/

Alta Vista, http://www.globalpromote.com/altavista.htm

And update your email signature and Social Networking profiles to include the URL of your new site.

SEARCH ENGINE OPTIMIZATION

Search Engine Optimization or SEO is a way of using keywords and phrases, the words people type into search engines, to direct traffic to your site and improve your rankings in search engine results.

This is a specialised area and it is easy to over-do the SEO words which can have a negative impact on your page rating. If you are using a web designer, ask for their advice. If you are doing your website yourself, keep the keywords down to a minimum.

Samples of SEO text include things like "if you are looking for a nail technician in Harrow..." Where two keywords have been merged: looking for a nail technician and nail technician Harrow.

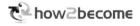

You can always take a free trial of some SEO software options to help you to find the correct keywords for your site.

Some suggested sites are: http://tizag.com/SEOTutorial/

http://www.jm-seo.org/seo-tutorial/google-keyword-tools.html

And http://www.seobook.com/

SOCIAL MEDIA – IS IT A WASTE OF TIME?

Come on, admit it, you know you've been thinking it, but in fact, social media is a really important way to get your business name known. This is why many companies suddenly have Facebook pages and Twitter accounts.

Being on Social Media can be an important part of your marketing plan, if, and it's a big if, you update your social networks regularly.

The fact is that many businesses use social media and social networks as a key part of their marketing campaign. If your potential clients are using social media, it only makes sense for you to be using it too, as this is yet another way you can come to your potential clients' attention.

Being active on social networks can:

- Increase traffic to your site

- Get your name into more networks, and raise awareness of your business

- Result in more clients finding your business

- Improve Search Engine Rankings which leads to higher page ratings in search engines, which could lead to more clicks to your site and more clients.

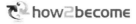 how2become

Make sure, however, that you are using social media as a vehicle to connect with potential clients and not just to spend loads of time chatting with friends and other nail technicians!

Don't randomly use social media. Schedule time in your diary when you will focus on 2 or 3 platforms such as Twitter, Facebook or LinkedIn and provide nail care tips and advice, or nail product reviews to your target markets so that you get well known and develop a following.

OFFLINE MARKETING STRATEGIES

Postcards
Prepare short marketing postcards informing clients of your services and how you can help them. If you're stuck on what to write then look at all the leaflets that come through your door and pick out the best points of each of them that attracts you to the advert. Stick to short phrases and bullet points for postcard advertising and ALWAYS include your prices. You can also offer a 50% off code or voucher on the card to attract clients to your business.

You can create your own postcards at Vista Print http://www.vistaprint.co.uk

Leaflets
You can go for A5 one sided leaflets or tri-fold leaflets advertising your services and your price list. Most local copy or print shops will design a leaflet for you based on your directions. Shop around as the prices per 1000 leaflets can vary considerably and yes you will need 1000s of leaflets if you are going to successfully market your business.

You need to do leaflet drops through the letterboxes of the homes of your target clients and not just once, but often two

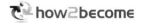

or three times at monthly intervals before your marketing pays off.

You can also enquire whether your local library, doctors' surgeries, schools, nurseries, dentists etc will let you put some leaflets on their tables too. This is a surprisingly good way to attract new clients as they have nothing else to do but read your leaflet – or the three year old copy of Reader's Digest!

Press Releases

A press release is a one page summary of your new business that sounds newsworthy. Local papers rely on press releases to help them fill the business news section.

You can either write a press release yourself, or hire a writer from a freelance site to write a press release about the launch of your new nail technician business and submit it to local newspapers and business magazines. If you are lucky, the paper might even interview you and put your photo in the paper too!

Word of Mouth

Word of mouth must be one of the most powerful ways in which to advertise your business. So drum up clients by making sure that everybody you know hears about it! Give them a copy of your price list and services sheets. This way they can pass the message on to their friends/family too. Friends, family and neighbours can be great testimonials and gain you valuable clients.

Referral Scheme

If an existing client recommends a new client, then reward your existing client by giving £5.00 off their next treatment.

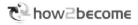

Other Marketing Tools You Could Use include

- Adverts in the local papers
- Adverts in shop windows
- Putting your business card on display in the local gym/ health club

ONLINE MARKETING STRATEGIES

Website

This is your ultimate selling tool. This needs to be professional looking and to sell your services 24/7 every day of the year. Do not rush your website. Every word you use on your website must count and will make an impact on your potential clients. Refer back to 'Setting up your Website' on page 59.

Your Emails

Design an email signature to attach to every email you send out to promote your nail technician business. You can create a professional looking marketing email at http://vistaprint.co.uk.

Social Media

Develop and regularly update a profile for your business on Facebook http://facebook.com, LinkedIn http://linkedin.com and Twitter http://twitter.com.

Blogging

If you are confident at writing, you could start up a blog to draw visitors to your website. Blog about being a nail technician, review new nail products, write a 'how-to' piece on something you are confident in doing, or blog about celebrity nails. Blogs can be set up for free at sites like WordPress.com (who will host your blog)

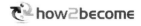

http://www.wordpress.com/ or you can use the WordPress blogging software on your own website by using http://wordpress.org. If you use http://www.wix.com you can add a 'blogging' widget to your website.

Write Articles for Sites/Magazines

Write an article about being a nail technician for your local paper, or write a guide on how to correctly file your nails, remove cuticles etc or why manicure parties are ideal or birthday party treats.

Remember, the purpose of blogging and article writing is to direct traffic (potential clients) to your website so always include your domain name.

Join Professional Organisations

It is worthwhile joining a professional organisation so that when people are looking for a nail technician in your area, they will come across you. Plus joining such an organisation gives you a support and information network too.

The only professional organisation in the UK for nail technicians is The Beauty Guild http://www.beautyguild.com but many find SalonGeek a very helpful forum for gaining advice and tips: http://www.salongeek.com/nail-geek.

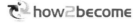

CHAPTER ELEVEN

CUSTOMER CARE

The first step in customer care is treating your client as if they are the most important person in the world. When a client comes for a treatment, they are concentrating on the 'treat' part of the word. They are looking for:

- Escape from the real word

- Pampering

- Conversation

- Attention

- Relaxation

- A sense of importance

So to keep your clients coming back make sure you remember this and treat them accordingly. They are looking for a beauty experience not just good nails.

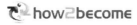

If you are working from home make sure:

- Your work area is welcoming, neat, tidy and professional looking
- It is relaxing and creates a 'spa' atmosphere
- You have everything you need to hand
- You can play some relaxing music

If you are a mobile technician then you need to ensure:

- You always arrive on time
- You have everything you need with you
- You set up your work space quickly and efficiently
- You help your client to relax and feel pampered.

Wherever you are working you also need to ensure that:

- You always look neat and professional (tunic, hair, make-up and nails)
- You always appear calm, relaxed and welcoming
- You look pleased to see them
- You remember their name and what you did for them last time.
- You don't chat on and on about your problems and life
- You don't gossip about other clients – they will worry you will do the same about them.
- You listen to your client – really listen and let them get their thoughts, worries or gossip off their chest.
- You talk to them
- Get customer feedback. Find out what they would like you to offer and take steps to offer it. Make your customers feel special and they will keep coming back to you.

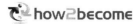

Client Records can help you to remember facts about your client. Ensure all your clients complete a record card so you have their name and contact details. You can use this card to note down the treatments they want done and what you do for them on each visit. You can also note down other 'facts' on this card to help you treat them as an individual.

You can buy client record cards online and from wholesalers, or you can keep an automated system.

DEALING WITH COMPLAINTS AND DIFFICULT SITUATIONS

It can be hard, very hard working with people. Sometimes people aren't always clear about what they want or sometimes they have unrealistic expectations. Some people, let's face it, are almost impossible to please.

If a customer complains do not get angry. It is hard to listen to what you might feel are unfair complaints face-to-face, but do not lose your temper. Remain professional, polite and take steps to remedy the situation.

Listen to what they have to say and take steps to resolve the situation calmly and to the customer's satisfaction.

Be assertive but not aggressive. If you are in the wrong, admit it freely. If it was a case of misunderstanding or poor communication – apologise and ask what you can do to put it right.

Take steps to remedy the situation before the client leaves. If you don't, they won't come back and remember, one complaint, repeated to enough people can soon have a detrimental effect on your business. So treat every customer as if they were your only one and you'll be fine.

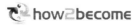

THE IMPORTANCE OF INSURANCE

As a nail technician either working in your own home or offering a mobile service to clients in their homes, you need to have insurance.

Most specialist providers of nail technician insurance provide this cover at a cost of around £40 per year.

This insurance will protect you if a client claims they were injured by you, your premises or your equipment. It also covers you for theft or loss of your products.

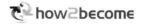

CHAPTER TWELVE

GAINING GREAT FEEDBACK

One of the best methods of marketing is when people recommend you to others. One way you can harness this is to ask your clients to give you feedback and ask for their permission to put this feedback on your website and in your marketing materials.

People respond better to client testimonials.

They are unbiased and seem more trustworthy than you just singing your own praises.

It is important, therefore to get positive client feedback and get it into your marketing materials as quickly as possible.

You could offer a draw for a free manicure for everyone who completes their feedback forms.

Or you could routinely ask you clients to complete a feedback

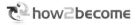

form or email you their comments. The easier you make it for people to give you feedback and the more methods you offer them to do so, the more feedback you are likely to get.

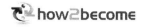

CHAPTER THIRTEEN

EXPANDING INTO OTHER AREAS

Once you have established your business as a nail technician, you might feel like adding extra services to your business and expanding into other related areas.

You can take extension courses at most local colleges and private health and beauty institutes.

For nail extension courses – such as air-brush or new techniques, it is a good idea to attend courses run by the manufacturers such as Bio Sculpture, Opi and Jessica Nails.

BECOMING A BEAUTY THERAPIST

Some nail technicians decide to expand into beauty therapy to widen their client base and the types of jobs they can do.

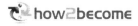

This is particularly recommended if you want to work on a cruise ship or in a holiday resort, health farm or spa.

You don't necessarily need to do a full NVQ course; you can, in certain areas, just take a course on the particular area of beauty therapy you are interested in such as

- Massage

- Hot Stone therapy

- Indian Head Massage

- Facials

- Waxing

To discover which courses are recommended by beauty therapists and which ones are most in demand, ask in the forums on SalonGeek.

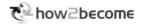

CHAPTER FOURTEEN

USEFUL RESOURCES FOR THE NAIL TECHNICIAN

TRAINING AND QUALIFICATIONS

British Association of Beauty Therapy and Cosmetology (BABTAC) http://www.babtac.com

Confederation of International Beauty Therapy and Cosmetology (CIBTAC), http://www.cibtac.com

Habia http://www.habia.org

International Therapy Examination Council (ITEC) http://www.itecworld.co.uk

VTCT http://www.vtct.org.uk

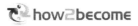 how2become

CODE OF PRACTICE, NAIL SERVICES, HABIA

http://www.habia.org/

INSURANCE PROVIDERS

The Beauty Guild: http://www.beautyguild.com

http://www.salonsaver.co.uk

http://www.professionalbeauty.co.uk

http://www.abtinsurance.co.uk/

PROFESSIONAL ORGANISATIONS AND RESOURCES

The Beauty Guild http://www.beautyguild.com/

Salon Geek/Nail Geek – forum for nail technicians with help and advice. http://www.salongeek.com/

Scratch Magazine – the magazine for nail technicians
http://www.scratchmagazine.co.uk/

Professional Beauty Magazine
http://www.professionalbeauty.co.uk/

Vitality Magazine (from BABTAC)
http://www.babtac.com/vitality-magazine/

NAIL TECHNICIAN JOB SITES

http://www.hair2beautyjobsource.com

http://www.indeed.co.uk/Nail-Technician-jobs

http://www.simplyhired.co.uk/a/jobs/list/q-nail+technician

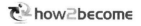

http://www.jobisjob.co.uk/nail-technician/jobs

http://www.gumtree.com/health-beauty-jobs/uk/
nail+technician+jobs

http://www.nailtechnicianjobs.org.uk/job-board

NAIL TECHNICIAN JOBS ABROAD/ON CRUISE SHIPS

http://www.leisurejobs.com/

http://www.onespaworld.com/

http://www.cruisejob1.com/

ACCOUNTING SOFTWARE

NCH Software http://www.nchsoftware.com/invoice/

QuickBooks http://www.intuit.co.uk/

SALON SOFTWARE

http://www.i-salonsoftware.co.uk

http://www.studiotracker.co.uk/

http://www.phorest.com/salonsoftwareuk

FREELANCE JOB BOARDS TO FIND WEB DESIGNERS, WRITERS AND LOGO DESIGNERS

Elance http://www.elance.com

Guru http://www.guru.com

ODesk http://www.odesk.com

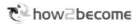

DOMAIN NAMES AND WEB HOSTING AND SETTING UP YOUR WEBSITE

Remember to choose a name that suits your needs and get a host that offers all the services you require. Look around before you buy.

http://order.1and1.co.uk/ this site offers .co.uk domains from as little as £2.49 a year, and .com domains from £6.99 a year. It also offers web hosting.

http://lcn.com/domain_names this site offers .co.uk domains from £3.00 a year, .com from £6.80 a year and .eu domains from 8 Euros a year.

http://123-reg.co.uk/ Offers domain names, web hosting and a variety of web hosting accounts.

http://fastvision.com/Domains.fvnx this site offers a vast array of domain extensions from .co.uk at £2.99 a year, but also .org, .net, uk.com and many, many more.

Browsershots enables you to see what your site looks like on all browsers. http://browsershots.org/

Get your site listed at Google, http://www.google.com/submityourcontent/

Alta Vista, http://www.globalpromote.com/altavista.htm

Yahoo and Bing (who now use the same submission service) https://ssl.bing.com/webmaster/SubmitSitePage.aspx

And for SEO help and advice, try the following sites:

http://www.tizag.com/SEOTutorial/

http://www.jm-seo.org/seo-tutorial/google-keyword-tools.html

http://www.seobook.com/

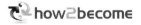

SETTING UP YOUR BUSINESS – ADVICE

Visit all of these sites for advice before taking the step to start up your own business; you might think this is a waste of your time, but it isn't. Time spent here is invaluable.

http://www.businesslink.gov.uk/

http://www.hmrc.gov.uk/

http://www.britishchambers.org.uk/

SOCIAL MEDIA

Develop and regularly update a profile for your business on

- Facebook http://www.facebook.com
- LinkedIn http://www.linkedin.com and
- Twitter http://twitter.com

FURTHER READING

The Complete Nail Technician (Hairdressing and Beauty Industry Authority) by Marian Newman (Paperback – 13 Apr 2011)

Encyclopedia of Nails (Habia City & Guilds) [Paperback]

A Complete Guide to Manicure and Pedicure [Paperback] by Leigh Toselli

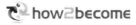

TREATMENT MATRIX WORKSHEET

Treatment	Qualified/ Skills/ Experience	Local Demand Yes/No	Do I want to offer this treatment?
Nail art			
Nail extensions			
Manicures – basic			
Manicures – luxury			
French manicure			
Japanese manicure			
Hot Oil Manicures			
Paraffin Dips			
Pedicures – basic			
Pedicures – luxury			
Gel wraps			
Acrylic extensions			
Nail repair			

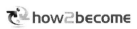

ACKNOWLEDGEMENTS

Our thanks go to the following nail technicians/beauty therapists for their contribution to this book.

Jo Cura	Beauty Therapist, Nail Technician and College Lecturer
Emma Briers	Nail Technician – Simply Nails
Danielle Cook	Salon Manager at Bare Beauty Salon
Isabella Hyde	Nails by Isabella

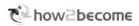

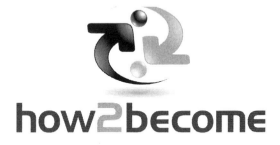

how2become

Visit www.how2become.co.uk
for more career guides and
resources to help you
be what you want.

www.how2become.co.uk